EFFORTLESS HEALING

The Easiest Way To Make Your Mind Resolve All Of Its Problems In Itself

I0449183

Written By

LAURA SERIO

ACKNOWLEDGMENTS

For my students and friends, who all selflessly helped me in writing this book. Special thanks to those who asked, insisted and assisted me in writing this book. I also like to give my deepest gratitude to my readers and friends who are reading all my books. All Rights Reserved 2012-2015 @ Laura Serio

TABLE OF CONTENT

INTRODUCTION

What would your reaction be if I tell you that just awareness of the problem can fix it? I know you say, "If I know my problem well, I can solve it with ease. There is nothing new about that."

If I say you have to do nothing and just become aware of the problem and it will be fixed in itself, what would you say? I am sure you would be amazed. Yes, awareness can do the fixing. If you notice the physical or mental problem like fear or anger, indigestion, failing relationship or headache, the organized part of awareness can do the fix. It isn't just shocking; it is wonderful. This skill can change your lifestyle in a very extraordinary way.

Awareness is the way to embrace your life which would enliven and soften the world where we live while healing your wounds, whether emotional, physical or mental. The awareness and healing force can be the solution of all your issues. This small book is all about healing effortlessly with the help of awareness.

Do you think you are aware? Is your brain conscious that you are reading and trying to understand these words? Are you aware what you are thinking just now? Are you are you are standing or sitting? By learning the easy steps in this book, you can heal your mind and body effortlessly.

In this book, you will also learn the ways to remove negative thoughts from your mind and the benefits of doing this. We are also discussing about effortless breathing techniques that will help you heal mental stress and help you feel the gap between your thoughts to improve your mind clarity. This book also contains some of the important questions you must ask yourself to know who you are and identify your real power.

CHAPTER 1

AWARENESS – THE VERY FIRST STEP OF HEALING YOUR MIND

Which thing or person you love the most in your life? Is it your job, family, spouse, children, health or your cute fluffy pet?

Ask this simple question to yourself and see how magically it changes the quality of your whole life. Keep reading and think about it properly.

The answer to this question is hidden in awareness. Awareness is the solution all your problems. You cannot work at your office with full energy, love your children and spouse to the fullest, or even enjoy the sidewalk or morning coffee without it. All your purposes and intents are nothing without awareness.

Awareness and mind are different things. If our mind is a light bulb, then awareness is electricity that supplies the power to it. Dull indication of awareness causes misunderstanding, confusion and even suffering to your mind. A bright mind with awareness is present and calm. It reflects peaceful gentleness to others. If awareness looks like "inner light" to you, then you are near your desire to understanding its value.

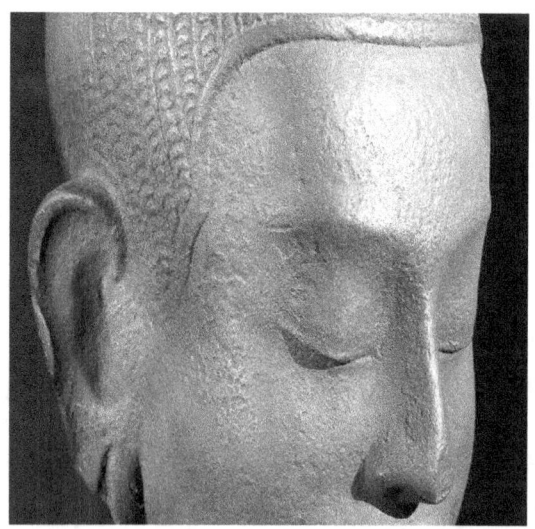

How Awareness Works?

How much you are aware shows how much the quality of your life improved. It is important to have awake and vibrant awareness in your life. Suppose you are locked in a room that is completely dark and light is trying to enter the room. When you look around and you keep watching little by little, and you will see that the room starts lightens and you start seeing the things more clearly.

All of a sudden, you see a snake is up to strike and you get scared. Your mind is loaded with fear and frantic thoughts – *will it attack if I move? Is the snake venomous? If it bites me, how would I seek help?* You are alone in the room and the light keeps on increasing and illuminating the area around you. Eventually, you start thinking clearly and your mind gets little relaxed and tries to analyze the ways to escape and your body is idle. When the sun summits the horizon, it releases the first rays and the dawn gets into the window and your room is filled with bright golden light. Then you realize that it is just a rope, not a snake.

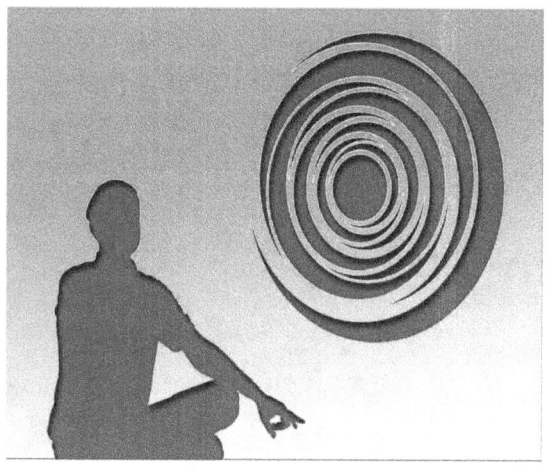

In those few moments, fear froze your mind and released thoughts that were sprinkled just like a broken glass. As a result, your tensed mind was releasing stress hormones and getting you ready to combat. During those moments, you felt the fear of threat that was nothing.

Impaired awareness is just like the darkness. Drug abuse, lack of exercise, overwork, unhealthy food habits, alcohol, greed, anger and grief diminish our awareness and keep us viewing the world consciously.

Our lives are full of threats which we have perceived unnecessarily. Here, we visualize the fear as snakes. In real life, we have job snakes, financial snakes, relationship snakes, and family snakes. Even when you are driving to a beach or movie, your mood can be upset with traffic jam which causes exploding temper and soaring blood pressure. In short, we are visualizing snakes all around in our world.

How Awareness Helps Improve Quality Of Life?

To improve awareness, we have to first kick off the snakes that are causing blindness and keeping us to see the world more clearly. We have to change our perceptions. You may consider awareness as a sunlight which enlightens our mind and lightens our emotions. Muddy emotions and dull minds are the evils of awareness. It is awareness that fuels up our perceptions and you can never be fooled by boneless fear if you have pure awareness.

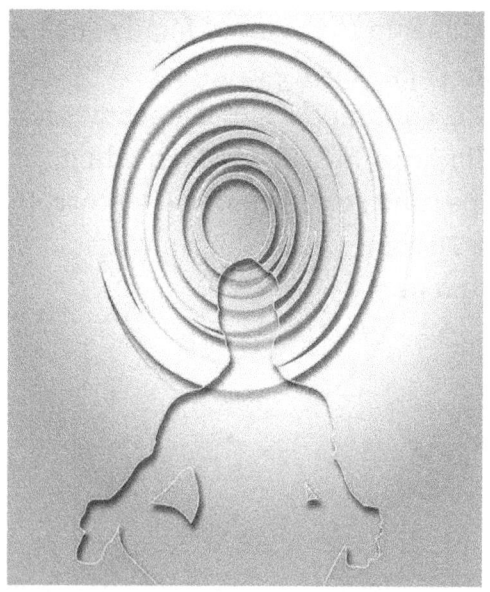

Our mind remains on "autopilot" mode most of the time. Our hyperactive mind wastes a lot of energy and cause troublesome situations. Some of the major symptoms of this problem are frustration, boredom, anxiety, anger, fear, worries about future, or thinking about the past. Due to dull awareness, our world starts looking like a dark or scary place and these ropes start looking like snake.

Awareness is around us every time and the best thing is that we don't have to think about it. Sounds weird? It is true! We are aware of people around and thoughts and stuffs in our life. Have we noticed awareness ever before? No, not really!!

In fact, many of us don't even notice when pure awareness walked up and helped us to make change. All in all, we don't have to notice awareness and understand it. All we need to have some knowledge about things. You may think of pure awareness natural, just like breathing. Pure awareness has no limits and it has no form that can be identified by our body. Our mind is the container of our emotions and thoughts.

CHAPTER 2

HEALING TOXIC THOUGHTS TO CALM OUR MIND

There is a factor which has more importance than any other in order to improve your health.

It worsens around 95% of your health if it is gone out of your life. It is very helpful to dramatically reduce the adverse effects of disease and increase longevity.

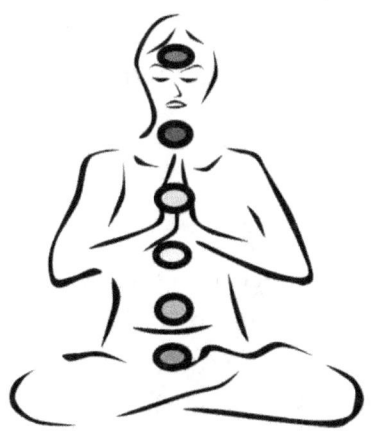

It also determines whether you would live healthier or longer life and it also includes considering blood sugar, cholesterol and blood pressure levels. But it cannot be found in doctor's office or doesn't come as a pill.

And that thing is your social networks, your attitude, your spiritual beliefs and your community. The healthy spirit and mind and the sense of connection to others can have great impact on your health. Along with healthy breakfast, the psychological resilience is another major factor for longevity. But there are some toxic thoughts that ruin our healthy lifestyle. Here are some tips to heal and transform your toxic thoughts and calm your mind down –

BREATHING

Let's start with one of the easiest ways to repair the toxicity in your emotions. Anyone can do this exercise. All you need to keep your hands on your heart and feel how it's moving while breathing. It feeds the energy of harmony, peace and love.

Look At Yourself

Before making any reaction to any challenging situation, try to see yourself in the mirror. There is no one who likes to see them reacting in negative way. Feels awkward? Don't stop yourself and don't take yourself too seriously.

Think Of Someone You Love The Most

In your emotions, the energy will go through all the living beings. If you have dealt with something which causes negative emotions to you, just think of someone you love or visualize their image. You might visualize the face of your beloved puppy, baby, kitten or your partner.

Watch Out Your Words

Your emotions, thoughts and words can change your experience and the world around you. It will work with both types of words – the words we talk to ourselves and the words we speak out loud. Suppose you admit that you are not a nice person, it will start showing it in real. So, have positive words in your mind and let your life to unfold it.

Reconnect With Nature

We all belong to nature. While we get stressed out, we get disconnected from the fostering we get from earth, fire, air and water and we become ill. But you can heal with the help of nature. Take time to connect with nature whenever possible.

Use Water

Water has life force that can easily clean off all your pain and can give you great healing effect. You can notice the negative energy going away from you when you take a shower, wash your hands or just stand in the rain.

Using Mind To Heal Your Body

You need to change how you perceive your body. A constant flow of information and energy appears to be a three dimensional object. Your body makes changes when it exchanges and shuffles its molecules and atoms with the world and you will do it faster than changing your outfits. Right now, your body is not in the same condition when you woke up or just a couple of minutes ago.

Our body has around 50 trillion cells that constantly interact with one another with which we digest our food and our heart can beat and our body can avoid toxins and prevent diseases and infections. Though these processes look out of control, there are hundreds of studies which proved that our mind is more powerful than our body.

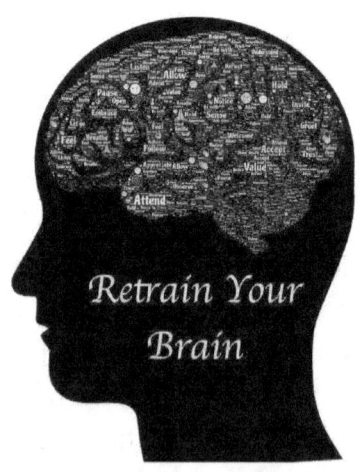

Neuropeptide is a molecule created by every emotion, feeling and thought that our mind develops. This molecule travels through the body and address the receptor sites of neurons and cells. Your brain receives this information and converts the same into chemicals and alerts the whole body if there is any reason for happiness or any trouble. Your body is directly connected to your mind and it sends the signal to our body that what you are feeling or thinking.

Suppose you say to yourself that you are upset, then you are actually upset. If you look inside, you will find that your body is affected by those molecules which cause damage or stress like huge amount of cortisol and adrenaline.

In order to use endless power of our mind, we need to increase the level of self-awareness. If awareness is distracted, the flow of information and energy around the mind and body is also distracted. You will likely to stay affected by toxic thoughts like resentment, regret and self-guilty. Inactive lifestyle and overeating also take toll of our body.

On the flipside, by expanding your awareness level, you will feel the free flow of energy. You will be more balanced, flexible and creative. You can have more energy to view the world around you with more understanding and compassion and you will be open to more new possibilities. There are several ways to increase your awareness like mindfulness and meditation. But here are other ways to help you out –

- **Be passionate about experiences you fill in your life**

- **Stay open to maximum input**

- **Be ready to make informed decision**

- **Work on your mental blocks like guilt and shame**

- **Be emotionally free**

- **Redefine yourself all day**

- **Don't scare of future and don't regret your past**

    Awareness directly helps you find the infinite power of your mind and create better health, love and happiness in life.

CHAPTER 3

HEALING MENTAL EFFORT & PAIN

Breathing is an important part of our life. The very first thing after birth and the last thing before death we all do is breath. In our whole life, we take breath around a billion times. Our body, mind and breath are intimately influenced and connected with each other. Our thoughts influence our breath and our breath is influenced by our thoughts. Breathing with awareness is very important to restore the balance between our body and mind. According to researchers, here are some benefits of deep breathing –

- Lower blood pressure
- Reduced depression and anxiety
- Muscle relaxation
- Increased energy levels

- Reduced feelings of overwhelm and stress

Deep breathing has positive impact both in our body and our mind. Most of these effects can be related to reducing stress response. Read on to know how deep breathing works.

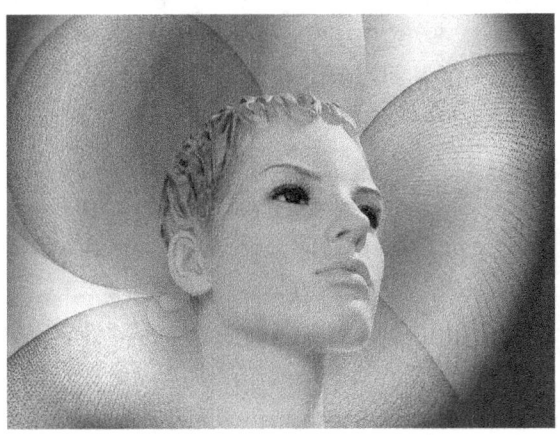

Breathing – The Effortless Way Of Healing Our Stress

When we feel stressful thoughts, it is our sympathetic nervous system that addresses the fight-or-fight response of our body and gives a burst of energy to react to the potential risk. Our breathing turns rapid and shallow and we basically breathe from upper body, not for the lungs. It can make us feel anxious and frustrated and we feel breath shortening due to it. At that time, the body forms a range of hormones like epinephrine and cortisol what boosts your pulse rate and blood pressure and keep us in state of high alert.

But you can avoid these problems dramatically and calm down your body and mind with deep breathing. By taking slow and deep breath, we turn on the parasympathetic nervous system to avoid stress in body. Deep breathing also arouse the main nerve in vagus nerve and control the blood pressure, calm down heart rate and please your mind and body. Deep breathing also helps engage diaphragm and abs muscles instead of upper chest and neck muscles.

Working with respiratory muscles improves oxygen exchange efficiency with every breath and allows more air exchange in lower lungs. It also reduces muscle strain on upper chest and neck and these muscles can relax properly. This way, deep breathing can cause more relaxing and calming effect and the tissues and cells of the body can get higher oxygen. Along with reversing stress response in your body, breathing exercises also slow and calm down the emotional stress. It can immediately diffuse the emotional energy.

Effortless Breathing Techniques For Self Healing

Along with the practice of deep breathing, there are several breathing techniques ancient yogis taught us who can have varied effect on our body and mind. The beneficial effects of breathing are also documented in curing

Posttraumatic Stress Disorder (PTSD), anxiety, depression, Chronic Destructive Pulmonary Disease (COPD), and asthma. Breathing can also help us improve longevity.

Virtually, all breathing techniques are based on the science of yoga. Pranayama is one of these breathing techniques. Pranayama refers to "Prana" which means life and "Yama" which means control. You can influence all parts of your life with breathing. You can improve your overall health by learning certain breathing techniques.

Complete Belly Breath

Relax your abs muscles by inhaling through your nose slowly and keeping one hand on belly. It will help you breath air directly to the bottom of lungs. You would feel abdomen rise and it will expand the lower lungs. Keep inhaling when your rib case expands and collar bones rise. Take a break for a while when you reach at the height of inhalation, and exhale gently from top to bottom of your lungs. Contract your abs muscles eventually to throw out the toxic air from the bottom of lungs when the exhalation ends.

Ocean's Breath

Try Ocean's Breath, also known as Ujjayi or cooling pranayama, if you feel irritated, angry or frustrated. It will calm and soothe your mind immediately:

- Take slightly deeper inhalation. Exhale through nose and constrict the throat muscles alongside. You would feel like the waves of ocean if you do it right.

- While exhaling, try listening to the sound "haaaaaah" while your mouth open to get hang of it.

Alternate Nostril Breathing

If you are feeling ungrounded or anxious, Alternate Nostril breathing is the best exercise to practice. It will cause immediate effect to calm your senses:

- Hold right thumb on right nostril and inhale through left nostril.

- When you reach the height of inhalation, use fourth finger to close the left nostril and lift right thumb and exhale with right nostril smoothly.

- After exhaling to the fullest, inhale with right nostril and close it with right thumb. When inhalation is done, close it with right thumb and exhale smoothly by lifting fourth finger.

- Keep practicing it for 3-5 minutes and alternate breathing with each nostril. Keep in mind that breathing must be easy and let your mind gently notice the outflow and inflow of breath.

Practicing deep breathing on regular basis is the best way to improve your overall well-being and health. Perform one of these techniques at least twice a day for 3 to 5 minutes to have long-term benefits. Whenever you feel stressed, practice one of these techniques at any time.

CHAPTER 4

HEALING EMOTIONAL STRESS

As compared to physical pain, emotional pain is more harmful for quality of your life. The negative emotions and stress related to any event can cause any disease or physical pain. Emotional stress is also associated to certain health problems like increased blood pressure, chronic inflammation, reduced immune response, raised tumor growth and distorted brain chemistry.

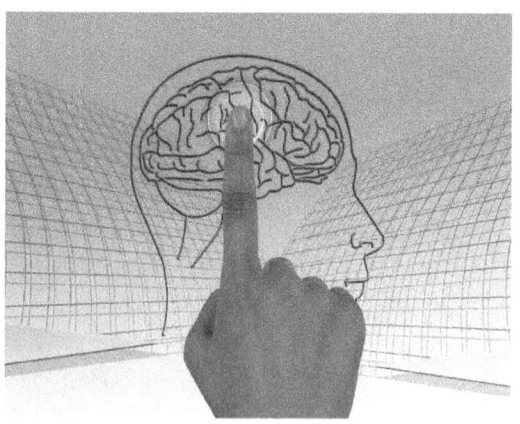

Emotional pain can also hinder your ability to live the life freely. Even worse, it may even make you wonder whether you are worth living your life.

Letting Go of Buried Emotions

Here are some of the practical strategies to cure rejection, guilt, and various psychological injuries that are associated to buried emotions -

Have You Got Rejection? Don't Lose Your Heart

Actually, rejection affects your brain in same way that physical pain does to your body. That's why it hurts that much. The feeling of rejection takes toll on your inner need of belonging and it hinders the ability to think, make decisions and recall memories. So, it is good to move on from these painful rejections for your mental health.

Stop Blaming Yourself

If you feel helpless after rejection or failure or blame it to your luck or lack of ability, it might affect your self-esteem. If you blame on specific things that were in your control like execution and planning, it might be less harmful. But it is better if you focus on alternative ways to improve yourself and be better prepared and informed to have better luck next time.

Guilt Can Be Useful

Guilt is like a "Relationship Protector" can keep you from doing something that can be harmful for another person. But excessive guilt can hinder your ability to concentrate and live the life to the fullest. After apologizing for anything, if you still are feeling guilty, make sure to express empathy to them and say that you know how your reaction caused impacts on them. It will likely help you relieve your feelings of guilt.

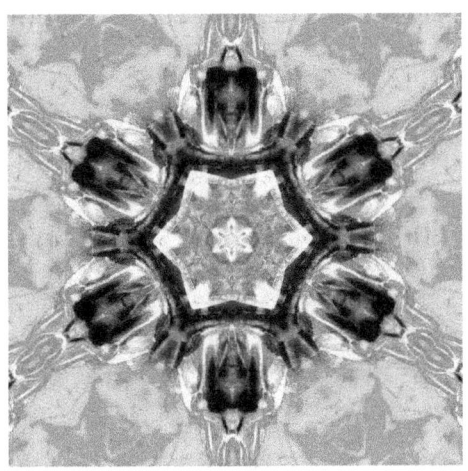

Why You Should Say "No" And How To DO It Politely?

Declining a project or invitation is difficult thing to do. But it doesn't mean you need to let the guilt rule your life or career.

"Good fences make nice neighbors." Everyone knows this. It means you should set firm boundaries. We need minimum unwanted interruptions and distractions and we want to have freedom to react the way we like. Especially in the age when people are desperate for attention and we have lots of ways to be distracted, it is really very important to make firm boundaries around us.

For both professional and personal growth, it is really very important to set boundaries and build firm fences. Ability to say "NO" is the vital part of good fence. We need to say "NO" to those engagements and activities that are not beneficial for us professionally and personally and that we don't like. Sometimes, we are afraid to say no to certain unwanted things and we end up saying "yes".

Especially for women, it is very hard to decline anything because they want to be liked. They like to come out as team players and they like to be the center of attraction. We don't like to hurt their feelings by declining their requests. We say "yes" to show that we can do everything.

Whatever the reason and whatever the story behind the scenes, one common thing is that saying yes to everything is counterproductive and overwhelming. If you say "yes" to a lot of things, you may ultimately be declining some of the things that are very important to you. If your plate is overloaded, you will not have any room for ideal or sudden opportunity. Everything will enter if you don't keep your fences strong.

So say yes, but only to those things that can help you advance your career or that you really enjoy, or which cannot distract you from your goals. Here's how to say "NO" politely and without feeling guilty –

Take a Pause for 24 Hours

Before saying yes to any proposal or invitation, whether personal or professional, take a pause for 24 hours. Don't reply back right away. Ask yourself if it is good to spend your valuable time over there, what you would get with it and if there is something you really like to do.

You may say "Thanks for inviting me. Let me think about it or check my schedule and I will tell you tomorrow". If you really like to do something but cannot do this time, just say "Thanks for the invitation. I cannot do this now but I would definitely do it in future and I hope you would remind me in future".

Say No Gracefully

Say No with authority and grace. We all can effortlessly say yes to anything but we cannot say no easily. If it's something we are not interested to do, we often try to find excuses. If you have got the invitation and you want to say no, do it gracefully yet authoritatively without guilt and excuses -

Try saying this if you want to decline invitation -"Thank you for such a great invitation. I'm afraid I cannot accept your invitation, but I appreciate your effort to including me." If someone forces you because of a reason, just say "I cannot just make it. But thank you very much." If someone really forces you, say, "I have a lot of things on pipeline. So, I will not be able to do it. Thank you."

CHAPTER 5

HOW TO EXPERIENCE THE GAP BETWEEN OUR THOUGHTS FOR BETTER MIND CLARITY

You may perhaps never have thought to have a space between the series of your thoughts and may not imagine it. Our thoughts hit our mind one by one. Sometimes, they overlap each other. We get thousands of thoughts every minute but can notice only 5 or 6 between them. So, how to mind the gap between these overlapping thoughts?

Just like every step you take, every thought we receive has a gap or space in between. You never think of it or you just get the thoughts without even noticing the gap. We can experience the gap between our thoughts and quiet our mind. Everyone suggests meditation to do every day for a reason. Meditation is the

most powerful part of life and it should
not be avoided.

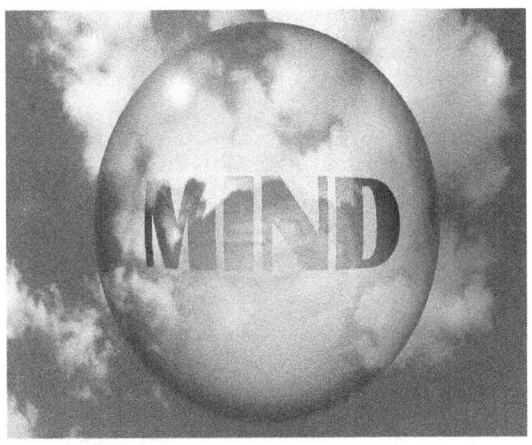

Our mind has been programmed to
stay active and work 24x7 and gets
thousands of thoughts in every minutes.
We cannot calm our body and mind if
they are on active mode. We are so busy
that we don't have time to discover
ourselves and find peace and silence in
the gap. This way, meditation is important
to calm and balance your mind. So, you
need to be take time to meditate for at
least 5 to 10 minutes. Believe it or not;

you will lighten and uplift your mind and calm your body.

The best thing is that meditation has no rules. All you need to sit quietly without movements and thoughts. Just try to notice the thoughts without judging them. Let them come in your mind.

Controlling Our Thoughts

It is possible to control your thoughts. There are destructive emotions that hinder the inner wisdom of our mind. Here are some of the helpful tips to control our mind and thoughts -

Make Plan for Your Life

Career, health problems and interpersonal desires are the part of our life, making it more complex than before. In cases of setbacks, negative emotions lead to sleepless nights and they adversely affect our health. So, get ready to change your life and make a plan to change whatever you want accept what you cannot change.

Practice Breathing

Practicing conscious breathing can calm down your body and control your emotions.

Let Positive Feelings Flow through Your Mind

If you feel annoyed, you cannot explore the beauty of something. But a relaxed body, plan for life and self-awareness will help you avoid negative emotions. A free mind will automatically see the beauty of life.

Accept that You Can Deal with Any Problem

Keep in mind that you can face any problem with positive thinking. Don't allow your problem distract your mind and solve it clearly.

Hear Good Music and Explore Good Things

This way will help you calm your mind and stay ready for positive thoughts. You can improve your focus if you listen to slow music and do some important thing alike. Seeing good sights can also help you stimulate your mind and let it think positive.

Bottom Line

Emotions can easily capture your mind and make you get struck with irrational logic. If work is not interesting, it is sure that you will feel tired, bored, and restless and lose focus. So, focus on your emotions if you want to get back to work smoothly. Emotions can block your mind from good thoughts. You determine to work hard every day but feel tired or bored. So, consider the symptoms of these emotions. Once you start focusing on a certain thing, it will drastically kill that feeling.

CHAPTER 6

WHAT IS QUANTUM HEALING?

There are some people who believe that our body is nothing more than energy. But the truth is that we are *conscious energy* that projects physical images. In fact, the whole universe is made of this conscious energy which is the core of everything. All of us are the essential part of this energy and it cannot leave us alone. It has all the intelligence and information of the universe.

Quantum healing adjusts or changes the electric fields to make changes in concept or idea. It neutralizes damaging or negative energies and their frequencies and treats them with more healing and harmonic perception. **Quantum Healing** is a natural process of healing which works with the energy of animals and humans.

How It Works?

Energy heal uses the subtle and deeper sources of energy like intention and thoughts to heal things. Subtle energy might sound weak but it is very powerful at atomic level. Thoughts don't feel much powerful at the initial level. But when your thoughts are combined with the thoughts of other people and focus the energy to heal something, it improves the healing process. This way, if both persons use the same energy to heal something, it can provide better results.

Several evidences have been found in quantum physics that prove that the major building blocks are formed with energy. According to them, intentions and thoughts can affect the behavior of energy. Since thoughts and intentions are responsible for that and everything is formed with energy, combining quantum healing with intentions and thoughts can heal our body deeply.

Unlike medicines, quantum energy is programmed to heal the deeper body structures. You can combine herbs and other holistic medicines with quantum energy techniques for better results. It will not just heal physical body, but also mind and soul.

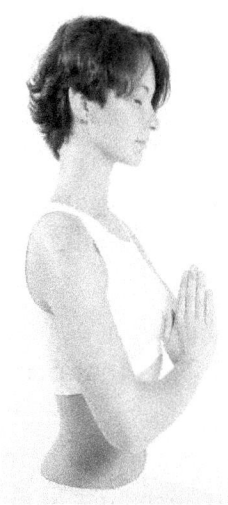

Why It Takes Longer Time to Heal Body with Quantum Energy

Using quantum healing techniques takes longer time than using conventional or holistic medicine to show results. Quantum healing addresses the body's energy structure which is found at deeper level than body's physical structures. Due to this reason, it needs longer time to show results.

This is why; most of us find it hard to trust quantum healing. We often like instant results because of which we switch to conventional medicines or herbs. But the problem is that any herb or medicine can repair your body at surface level. Quantum healing is more effective because it heals in deeper level.

Quantum Healing Techniques To Fix Body, Mind And Soul

Acupuncture

It is an ancient art of healing which stimulates the flow of energy and gets it back to normal state in your body. In this therapy, needles are calmly inserted in your skin at certain acupoints to improve energy levels in your body. Acupoints or acupuncture points are small centers of electromagnetic energy in our body.

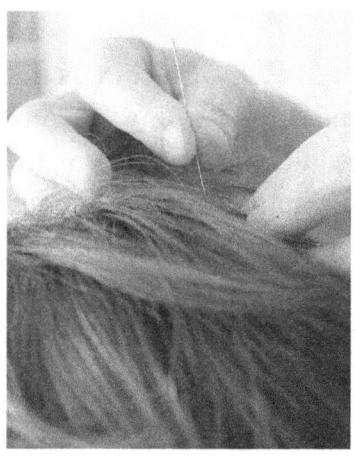

Crystal Healing

Crystals are known to transport the thoughts and energy and can be used as a mode to transfer the healing frequency. Crystals are known to be the best part of healing subtle energy as they can effectively amplify the power of frequency. Scientists who studied the connection between frequency and disease know the power of frequency for healing body.

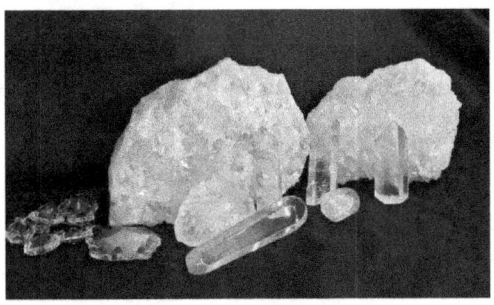

Reiki

It is a Japanese art of healing which uses life force energy to repair your body. It is a healing technique that uses spiritual energy to repair your body.

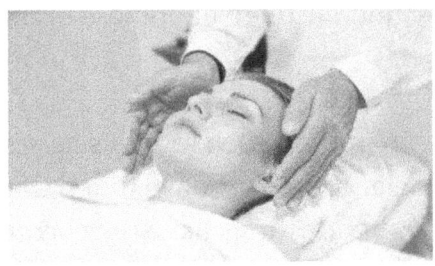

CHAPTER 7

GETTING TO KNOW YOURSELF

Almost all of us know that we have to know ourselves first to achieve anything in life. We all have hidden talent to develop innovative things and get prolonged happiness.

Problem is that most people don't just start knowing about themselves and figure out their hidden potential. We are mystified so deeply that we keep floating around low self-confidence and overconfidence. In one moment we find a unique purpose of life and, in the next minute, we get completely isolated. How can we find ultimate happiness in that case?

In my research to find self-growth, purpose and clarity, I have found that some right questions have the correct solution for our life. Here are some of the ideal questions to ask your mind and get started on the voyage of finding yourself and unearth the hidden potential for lasting happiness.

Questions To Ask Yourself To Help You Unlock Your Hidden Potential

What Makes You Stand Out and Be Special?

We all have something unique in this world. We cannot find the exact replica of ourselves here. Stop thinking of what you don't have, what others want from you, what you want to be, for a while. Think about the one thing makes you unique. Acknowledge what you have "special" and respect it.

How Do People See You?

Do they see the special person in you? Do people like your special abilities? If not, why and how to change it?

"We judge ourselves with our abilities; others judge us with our achievements."
~Henry Longfellow

This quote may help you to find the answer. How would you fill the space between what you really are and what you can be?

If money was not your problem, what would you like to do the most?

Become a singer? Write a book? Spend some time with loved ones? Or raise a serene garden? Don't limit yourself to daydream. Take your time. After having a vision, figure out the very first step which is easy and help you get a step ahead to your vision. Once you start working on your vision, the world will help you make it real.

What Would You Like to Do and What You Really Are?

There's nothing complex in this question and it is as easy as it seems. Suppose you say "You are an engineer but you have always wanted to become a writer." You can figure out the ways to connect both. You may create your own tech blog or write your own eBook about engineering.

What Makes You Feel Grateful?

Just think about the friends and family you have, your ability to hear, see, talk and walk, and try to be grateful because millions of people in the world who don't have such things. Did you hear the well-known saying – "I cried because I didn't have shoes until I met someone who doesn't have feet."

If you're going to die Next Day, Would You Be Feeling Satisfied with Your Past Life You Lived?

Figure out how you lived your life before? Do you have good memories that will last for lifetime for family? Have you apologized to everyone with whom you have done wrong or forgiven all of them who have done something wrong to you?

What's The One Movie that is Close to Your Heart and You like Watching Again and Again?

Our mind is designed to respond to narratives strongly. The story that tells you the most about yourself may touch you the most. What's the movie you would like to watch again and again?

If you are On a Ship that is sinking with All Your Acquaintances and You Could Save Only 10 People, Who Would They Be?

Most of us don't realize who we give most importance in our lives. We often try to attract random people who barely care about us and avoid those who matter the most. Do you know some people who really are important to you? Are you doing well to them?

Bonus Question

What would your life be after reading the above points? Would you just keep going like before while whining and arguing things the way with the people around? Or, will you live your life the way as it is a treasure and enjoy every small moments in your life?

DISCLAIMER

No part of this publication is allowed to be reproduced or copied by any photographic, mechanical, or electronic means, as photographic recording or scanning. It is not intended to be transmitted, stored in any system or be copied for personal or public use, without written permission from the author and the publisher.

The author doesn't recommend any medical suggestion or prescribe any kind of technique for treating emotional, physical and mental problem without the consent of a professional, either indirectly or directly. The book is published with the intention to provide only general information to cope up with spiritual and emotional stress. If you implement any idea from this book in your real life, both author and publisher shall not be responsible for any loss or harm.

ABOUT AUTHOR

I am Laura Serio, a writer by profession. After completing my graduation I got married and started writing books at home. I always wanted to inspire and help people with my writings. So, I started writing books on Health, Fitness & Dieting niche. My first book was "Natural Body Scrubs At Home", which contains homemade ideas to make scrub after that I wrote the next book on "Essential Oils For Beginners", it has so many healing remedies from essential oils an aromatherapy. After that I wrote a few other books, namely, "Natural Body Detox", "Carb Cycling", "Yoga For Beginners" and now the latest one is "Effortless Healing". All my books are related to health, fitness and dieting. More are coming soon. Follow me to get recent updates from me about my newly released books.